"In his compelling book on borderline person_____ ___ (BPD). Daniel Fox offers a profound understanding of this _____ with practical strategies for navigating its cha_____ and empathy, he sheds light on the nuances _____ to cultivate resilience and foster healthier _____ resource is a beacon of hope for individuals with BPD and their loved ones, and I will be regularly signposting my patients to this brilliant book."

—**Mark Silvert, MBBS, MSc, MRCPsych, MD,**
    consultant psychiatrist and medical director at the Blue
    Tree Clinic in London, UK

"This guided journal is an invaluable resource for individuals grappling with BPD. Daniel Fox's expertise in treating BPD equips him with the profound ability to pinpoint the core issues associated with this disorder and offer tangible, self-directed skills. Serving as a perfect complement to a holistic therapeutic approach, this guided journal is poised to make a meaningful difference in the journey toward managing BPD."

—**Liz Ross, PhD**, clinical psychologist, owner of the
    Coping Resource Center, and president of the Houston
    Psychological Association

"Daniel Fox's journal is the ideal marriage of research and practical utilization, providing readers with an evidenced-based approach to identifying and expressing their feelings, embracing self-acceptance, and gaining control of their inner struggles in a self-guided fashion. *The BPD Guided Journal* encompasses the broad areas of BPD, while providing tools for focusing on the reader's unique needs and goals, and is sure to make a difference in the lives of many people."

—**Jenna Turner, PsyD, ASOTP**, licensed psychologist in Texas
    specializing in clinical and forensic psychological assessment
    and treatment of at-risk youth with trauma-involved emotional
    and behavioral disturbances

"Whether you're someone coping with BPD or a mental health professional working with BPD clients, this journal is an indispensable resource. Fox has masterfully crafted a direct and easy-to-follow approach to help navigate the challenges that come with BPD. With this journal in your hands, you can feel confident you'll have the tools necessary to feel empowered to make real progress toward your future."

—**Kimberly McFarland, MS, LPC, NCC, ACS, CAADC, CDBT**, founder and therapist at the Therapy Institute of Michigan and Evolution Mental Health Services

"This book is an amazing resource that serves as a guiding light to help navigate the journey through BPD by illuminating pathways toward self-understanding, overcoming obstacles, and envisioning a better future. Readers discover strategies to manage symptoms while fostering resilience and self-compassion through engaging journaling exercises. With its accessible style and informative content, *The BPD Guided Journal* emerges as an indispensable companion for clients and great resource for clinicians."

—**Diane Stoebner-May, PhD, ABPP**, associate director and training director of the Sam Houston State University Counseling Center in Huntsville, TX

"One of the most challenging facets of BPD is the sentiment that meaningful, lasting improvement is impossible. Fox's book challenges the reader to push past self-doubt and curate confidence in their ability to navigate their experience with the disorder. This self-directed resource, crafted through a lens informed by decades of experience with personality disorders, empowers the reader to be their own advocate in their journey to mental health."

—**Tennille Warren-Phillips, PsyD**, founder of Relate Psychological Services, a private practice specializing in the diagnosis and treatment of personality disorders

New Harbinger Journals for Change

Research shows that journaling has a universally positive effect on mental health. But in the midst of life's difficulties—such as stress, anxiety, depression, relationship problems, parenting challenges, or even obsessive or negative thoughts—where do you begin? New Harbinger *Journals for Change* combine evidence-based psychology with proven-effective guided journaling techniques to help you make lasting personal change—one page at a time. Written by renowned mental health and wellness experts, *Journals for Change* provide a creative and safe space to process difficult emotions, work through challenges, reflect on what matters, and set intentions for the future.

Since 1973, New Harbinger has published practical, user-friendly self-help books and workbooks to help readers make positive change. Our *Journals for Change* offer the same powerfully effective tools—without ever *feeling* like therapy. If you're committed to improving your mental health, these easy-to-use guided journals can help you take small, actionable steps toward lasting well-being.

For a complete list of journals in our *Journals for Change* series, visit newharbinger.com.

THE
BPD

Guided Journal

Your Space to Release Intense Emotions,
Nurture Self-Compassion,
and Take Charge of
Borderline Personality Disorder

DANIEL J. FOX, PHD

New Harbinger Publications, Inc.

Publisher's Note

This publication is designed to provide accurate and authoritative information in regard to the subject matter covered. It is sold with the understanding that the publisher is not engaged in rendering psychological, financial, legal, or other professional services. If expert assistance or counseling is needed, the services of a competent professional should be sought.

NEW HARBINGER PUBLICATIONS is a registered trademark of New Harbinger Publications, Inc.

New Harbinger Publications is an employee-owned company.

Copyright © 2024 by Daniel J. Fox
New Harbinger Publications, Inc.
5720 Shattuck Avenue
Oakland, CA 94609
www.newharbinger.com

All Rights Reserved

Cover design by Amy Shoup

Interior Design by Tom Comitta

Acquired by Elizabeth Hollis Hansen

Edited by Amber Williams

Printed in the United States of America

26   25   24

10   9   8   7   6   5   4   3   2   1   First Printing

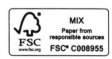

This journal is dedicated to my three heartbeats:
my wife Lydia and my two children, Alexandra and Sebastian.

It is also dedicated to New Harbinger Publications,
who continue to champion my intrinsic desire to bring
clarity and understanding of borderline personalty
disorder to those who need it the most.

Contents

Part 2: Surmounting Obstacles to My Growth

Part 3: Paving My Empowered Future

How Will This Journal Help Me?

This journal is designed for you, a person with borderline personality disorder (BPD) or BPD traits, to offer you not only a helping hand to get through the days but also ways to develop the inner strength that'll help you take on your BPD and tell it how you're going to live, as opposed to it always telling you. This journal will fully embrace my mantra:

Knowledge Is Empowerment

We're going to tap into your core content: those issues, beliefs, emotions, images, and so on that perpetuate your BPD and strengthen it and push you down the road of self-destruction. We'll also directly address the maladaptive behaviors and patterns that disrupt your life, the choices you make, and the choices you could make to build a life in which you, not your BPD, are running the show.

You may feel that your BPD has you wrapped in chains, but it's time to break free!

There's Real Hope

Much of the current view of BPD is outdated. BPD used to be seen as an "untreatable disorder," but research shows that this old belief is false—a reality that the mental health community needs to embrace more fully. The research shows that 50 percent of individuals with BPD achieve recovery—defined as the remission of symptoms and having good social and vocational functioning during the previous two years—from BPD. But wait, there's more: 93 percent of individuals with BPD attained a remission of symptoms lasting at least two years; 86 percent attained a sustained remission lasting at least four years; and of those who achieved recovery, only 34 percent relapsed—which, when looked at another way, means 66 percent *didn't* relapse (Gunderson et al. 2011; Zanarini et al. 2005).

So, this disorder is not simply a 10,000-pound cinder block around your neck. It may feel that way sometimes, but hope, insight, and skill-building will help you manage those thoughts, emotions, and behaviors that adversely impact your relationship with yourself and others.

You're Not Alone

One of the best aspects of therapy is having someone who is nonjudgmental and cares about your growth and wellness. This is something I strive for with all my clients. In this journal, I want you to feel that it's you and me, walking side by side, contending with those issues that pertain to your BPD in the past, present, and future.

Journaling is a powerful tool. It's for exploration but it's also an opportunity to push back on those fears, thoughts, and images that have kept you linked to your BPD. This journal is built on the work from my previous publications, *The Borderline Personality Disorder Workbook*, the *Complex Borderline Personality Disorder* book, and *The BPD Card Deck*; it's effectively the amalgamation of my approach. It also perfectly serves the goals of building insight and creating strategies to help you manage your BPD issues, instead of your BPD issues managing you. We'll also work to help you build your self-compassion through the journaling process.

A Map for the Journey

This journal is going to take you through three separate but related phases of growth to help you break free from your BPD. These three phases are:

1. Discovering Who I Am and Where I'm Going

2. Surmounting Obstacles to My Growth

3. Paving My Empowered Future

"Discovering Who I Am and Where I'm Going" is the initial phase of the journal and provides you with opportunities to recognize the influence you have on both your life and your perspective of yourself. The activities will promote self-discovery and insight building and teach you foundational skills to manage the four elements of BPD: emotions, thoughts, behaviors, and relationships (with yourself and others). As you'll see from the figure on the following page, these elements impact and reinforce one another. That's what can make the core of your BPD thoughts, feelings, and behaviors hard to control—but, crucially, it's not impossible to intervene in the cycles that can form between the elements, if you understand how they relate to one another.

The Four Elements of BPD

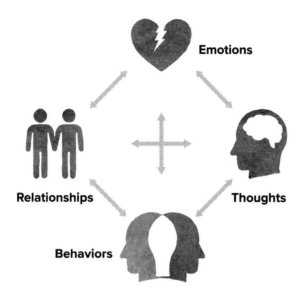

Emotions

Relationships

Thoughts

Behaviors

In the second section of the journal, "Surmounting Obstacles to My Growth," we build on the skills and insight you gained in phase one. We'll look into your BPD beliefs, behaviors, and self-destructive patterns while building your motivation to respond differently to yourself and others.

Finally, "Paving My Empowered Future" is the last part of the journal, but not of your journey. In this phase, we're going to build on the insight you'll have gained in previous sections by connecting your present with your desired future. This will include learning to continue to use the four elements of BPD to visualize a future of greater emotional control, more stable relationships, and nurtured self-compassion and acceptance.

Ultimately, each activity in this journal will tap into at least one of the four elements. Each entry will address one of the symptoms related to the four elements to help you not only focus on a particular aspect of your BPD but also to increase your insight into which larger element of BPD you're addressing. And the three phases of the journal, combined with the four elements of BPD, will help you move along on your journey to control your BPD and break free from its hold over your life. It's possible, and this journal can be a critical impetus to that freedom.

How to Use This Journal

Use this journal daily, weekly, or when you want. The more you use it, the more insight and strategies it will provide for you and the more often and instinctively you'll be able to replace maladaptive and self-destructive strategies with adaptive and empowering ones.

You can go through the journal in a linear fashion, from page one until the end. You can also jump to activities centered on the specific elements that cause you the greatest concern at this time, such as relationships. This journal is static but flexible, as it's designed to grow with you and can be molded into a variety of ways to fit your needs. You can also revisit already-completed exercises as issues arise at various times in your life. For example, say you have issues with your BPD-related thoughts and emotions when you start a new job or begin working with a new therapist. You can revisit the activities centered on these aims, even if you've completed them previously.

In the end, however you decide to work with it, this journal will help you build insight and skills. You'll learn to build emotional permanence, create strengthening affirmations, practice self-acceptance and gratitude, reduce guilt and shame, and more.

It's time to embark on this journey together and explore, grow, and empower you to break free from your BPD.

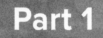

Part 1

Discovering Who I Am and Where I'm Going

What My BPD Looks Like

You may think you know the degree that the BPD elements impact you, but until you assess it, it's hard to know for sure. Using the boxes below, color in the degree of impact each element has on you today. For example, if your emotions have a severe impact on how you see yourself, others, and your world, color that column in up to the "Severe" level.

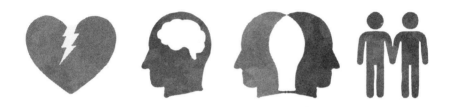

Emotions	Thoughts	Behaviors	Relationships
Extreme	Extreme	Extreme	Extreme
Severe	Severe	Severe	Severe
Moderate	Moderate	Moderate	Moderate
Mild	Mild	Mild	Mild
Absent	Absent	Absent	Absent

Goals for My Journey

Write out what you hope and want out of using this journal. These goals may change, and that's okay. Goals are not concrete, they're fluid.

The Purge

Emotions are better out than in, in many cases. Problems arise when we act on those emotions, harming ourselves or others. Releasing your emotions to a safe place can help you, particularly by writing them out in any way you want—tiny, huge, jagged, tight, and orderly, and so on. In the emotional purge box below, let 'em rip.

The Who and Why in My Life

Taking stock of the people in your life, the quality of those relationships, and what makes them that way is a very empowering and insight-building exercise. Describe the top three people in your life, the quality of those relationships (close, distant, estranged, and so on), and what makes them that way.

1st	2nd	3rd

Scaring Myself

Many people with BPD are afraid of their own behavior, and because of this, they don't explore it. Describe what aspects of your behavior scare you and what you could do differently.

From Where I Was to Where I Am

Identify three aspects of your life where you've grown and provide at least one clear example for each below.

1st	2nd	3rd

Impulse Without the Action

Living with BPD is formidable. BPD can drive you to respond automatically when you're stressed or angry, or act out in self-harm, without even thinking about the consequences. Describe those sensations, thoughts, and behaviors that trigger your self-harm impulse and what healthy behavior you can put in its place.

Emptiness to Fullness

You can go from emptiness to fullness through building your awareness. In the left column below, write what encourages your emptiness, and in the right column, describe what helps you feel full.

What Encourages My Emptiness	What Helps Me Feel Full

Your Relationship Value

Describe what you bring to relationships that makes them positive and unique.

Meditation Mantra

Lay down and get comfortable. Give yourself two to three minutes to just focus on you and the skills you have that help you move forward and manage your BPD beliefs, behaviors, and patterns. Mold these skills into a mantra.

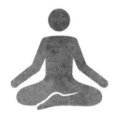

Mantras can help you think clearly, encourage growth, and know yourself more honestly.

For example, if you have insight into your thoughts and feelings, you could say to yourself, "My wisdom of self empowers me to choose for myself." Write your mantra below:

Disconnected to Connected

Let's recognize those things that help you feel detached from and attached to others in your life.

Describe what encourages your feelings of disconnection from others:

_____

_____

_____

_____

Describe what helps you feel connected to others:

_____

_____

_____

_____

_____

Feelings to Habits

Habits are created by our responses over time; this includes our responses to our feelings. Building awareness helps us control them—and journaling is a great way to build awareness.

Write your strongest feelings and the habits associated with them (for example, "anger" and "lashing out"):

_____

_____

_____

_____

_____

_____

_____

_____

_____

But wait, there's more… Check out the "Behaviors to Habits" exercise on the next page!

Behaviors to Habits

Taking the next step from feelings to habits, describe the feelings you want to strengthen, and what you can do to make them habits (for instance, "calm" and "planning my response").

(The secret is practice, practice, practice. Consider what opportunities you might have to practice the behaviors you just wrote down.)

Why I Fear Abandonment

Describe what makes abandonment so frightening for you.

_____

_____

_____

_____

Many abandonment fears lead to relationship disruption. Write how your fear of abandonment causes problems in your relationships.

_____

_____

_____

_____

Pushing Back on Abandonment Fears

Using what you wrote in the previous entry as a guide, what can you do to decrease relationship disruption associated with your abandonment fears? For example, describe how you can be more patient and listen more fully.

What Does Abandonment Really Mean?

Describe here what the end of a relationship means to you, then write what words of encouragement would help you feel better.

Embrace Your Awesomeness

Make a list of attributes that make you special and a worthy partner to be with or a worthy friend or family member to have. Take note of how you feel after you've made your list.

Presenting Your True Self

Describe how you can present your true self to your partner (or to future partners, if you're not in a relationship). Your true self is made up of those thoughts and feelings that make you **YOU**. To help, ask yourself, "Who am I really?"

Acting First, Thinking Second

Describe an instance when you acted first without thinking, and regretted it later.

_____

_____

_____

_____

_____

Write out your plan to do it differently next time.

_____

_____

_____

_____

_____

The next time a similar situation comes up,
see if you can put this plan into practice.

Swimming Thoughts

People with BPD tend to have negative thoughts on repeat swimming through their head, which empowers their BPD. Write out the thoughts that often swim in your head. Then rewrite them as positives, in a way that empowers you, not your BPD.

Hope over Emptiness

Many individuals with BPD experience intense feelings of emptiness that shroud their hope. Define or draw how your hope can empower you beyond your emptiness.

Partner Unsplitting

Think back to the last time you split on your partner—seeing them as all good or all bad, as opposed to the mixture of positives and negatives that we all are. What were those extreme, black-or-white thoughts? Write them below, then replace the extreme terms with more neutral or supportive ones—changing "must" or "always," for example, to "maybe" or "could be."

Impulsive Self-Destruction

Individuals with BPD tend to engage in self-destructive behaviors. Write about your top two—and what you could do instead next time you get the urge.

Self-Protective Sources

What are the things you can do to keep yourself safe and feel supported? Many people use images, like those below, to help remind them of healthy sources of safety.

Emotional Time Bomb

It's common for folks with BPD to feel like ticking time bombs because they're holding in their emotions. What if you managed your emotions differently? Below, write down your time-bomb emotions, then how you can get them out in an adaptive way (for example, exercise, scream, sing out loud, and so on).

Time-Bomb Emotion	Adaptive Release

When I Overvalue You

It's common to overvalue someone you just met and get enraptured with them and lose your sense of self. Write out those thoughts and emotions you often feel when you first meet someone. Recognizing your thoughts and emotions helps you control them, instead of them controlling you.

Say "No" to Fight Club

When you have BPD, impulsive behaviors and the urge to fight someone (or yourself) can rise quickly inside you. Acting out in these moments tends to lead to regret and loss later. List those things you can do instead of joining Fight Club next time you get the urge.

Undoing Regrets

All of us have regrets, including those with BPD and without, but we have to forgive ourselves for past mistakes and move on. List your top three regrets and then write a note of forgiveness to yourself.

1. ....

2. ....

3. ....

I forgive myself for:

Meaning of Rejection

Individuals with BPD are often highly sensitive to rejection. Describe what rejection feels like for you and what you can do to encourage self-acceptance and support when these feelings arise.

Partner Secrets

It's common for people with BPD to be afraid to reveal their true emotional self out of fear of rejection. Due to this, many do not tell their partners what they wish their partners knew about them. Write out what you wish your partner (now or in the future) knew about you. This is the first step to revealing your true self.

That Foodie Feeling

Many individuals with BPD struggle with food and with overeating to feel full. This is an attempt to combat that feeling of psychological emptiness.

Describe your psychological feeling of emptiness and fullness after an eating episode. Push back against self-condemnation, if that instinct arises; use an objective lens or a self-compassionate one.

My BPD-Biased Brain

Mind reading (when you assume what someone else is thinking without having much overt evidence) is a common protective strategy to keep you from getting hurt, but it leaves you open to the bias of your BPD. Describe how you might've used mind reading today and with whom, and keep an eye out for that BPD bias in the future.

Your Emotional Powder Keg

A powder keg of emotions pertains to a situation so full of feelings and triggering content that you feel you may explode into violence. Writing it out helps you release it in a healthy way. Consider a recent situation that left you feeling like a powder keg of emotions. Describe the what, when, and why of the situation that lit the fuse. Don't forget—swear words are ideal here!

Ringing My Abandonment Alarm

Relationships can be very scary, especially if you feel you don't know or trust yourself. Because your abandonment alarm is on autopilot, you likely find that you react after your alarm is ringing without you really knowing what's caused it. Describe those situations and people that tend to ring your alarm, and what it feels like when it's about to ring.

All of It Always

Overgeneralizing is when you assume something from one event, person, behavior, and so on to all others that are similar. For example, "My boyfriend cheated on me, so all guys cheat." List some of your overgeneralizing assumptions below to build your awareness of this cognitive distortion.

Tsunami of Sadness

Sadness can be overwhelming, confusing, and all-encompassing. This is part of what makes it hard to control. When you describe your sadness and understand what's caused it, you're empowered with insight. Describe your tsunami of sadness in as much detail as you want. Then, include one or two things that give you joy to turn that tsunami into a ripple.

The Power of Love

Love is linked to the hope of connecting to another person. Describe the things that add to and detract from you building and having hope in one of your current relationships. This can be any relationship—with a partner, parent, sibling, friend, coworker, and so on.

Drinking and Drugs

Substance abuse is a common comorbid condition that complicates BPD, and it lowers the probability of successful treatment. Circle the things below that add to your difficulty with drugs and alcohol to help you build insight into those contributing issues.

Fear

EMPTINESS

Self-hatred

Loneliness

Anger

Pain from
past abuse

Rejection sensitivity

Parent(s) abused
drugs & alcohol

FRIENDS USE

Not knowing who I am

Hopelessness

Abandonment fears

**An avoidance
coping style**

Chronic pain

Socially Isolated

Seeking excitement

ONGOING
STRESS

The world sucks

Pulled Toward Drinking and Drugs

Consider some of the items you circled on the previous page. How do these contributing issues manifest in your day-to-day life? Do you find you use in certain especially stressful moments or experiences? Take some time to write about your experience here.

Awareness Without Control

Your BPD drives those maladaptive beliefs, behaviors, and patterns that you think you have no control over. Build some awareness now by teasing out those you *can* control from those you can't.

Can Control	Can't Control

Depressive Spirals

A depressive spiral is a feeling that you're down, sad, unmotivated, and disheartened that lasts for less than one week. These spirals are common in those with BPD. Describe your last spiral, what caused it, how long it lasted, and how it was resolved.

Listening Without Hearing

Remember those times when someone gave you a response that made you feel unheard? They told you, "It gets better," "Everyone feels that way," or "It'd be easier if you weren't so emotional," and so on. Describe what statements help you feel heard and understood. Then tell those important people in your life because they may not know.

Your Social Disconnect

BPD can amplify the feeling of being excluded or ignored, which can cause you to act in a manner that adds to being socially detached. Identify those behaviors that encourage social connection and those that drive estrangement.

Connection   **Estrangement**

My False Self

We all have a false self to varying degrees. This is a facade or mask that you create to protect your true, authentic self, and it is often created and maintained by fear and doubt. BPD amplifies your belief in your false self, which adds to the confusion about who you are and what you believe. Your true self is that genuine part of you without the distortion of your BPD. Describe what your false and true self say to you in the following two conditions.

When I see myself in the mirror:

False self:

True self:

What type of romantic partner I am:

False self:

True self:

Fear of Losing *You*

BPD is intense and it can cause you to fear losing control, even before something happens to trigger you. Describe that feeling of losing your emotional self-control and what you're afraid might happen, then end with an encouraging statement to yourself.

Encouraging statement:

What Is Love?

All of us are looking for a loving relationship that helps us feel safe and understood. Identify those traits and behaviors in others that help you feel seen, secure, and heard.

The Light-Switch Myth

There is a false belief that managing BPD and your behaviors is as easy as flipping an on-off switch. If only it were that simple! In the space below, describe what "flips your switch" on and off: what helps you maintain your behavioral control, and what often drives you to lose it.

On

_____

_____

_____

Off

That Thriving Thought

If you could go back in time and tell the younger you to replace a toxic thought that would have made today a better day, what would it be?

And if you were to replace a toxic thought with a more balanced, adaptive, and helpful one now, what would it be?

How Emotionally Aware Am I?

If we can't recognize it, we can't control it. Take a moment and scan your mind and body. Then mark which of the six most common emotions you're feeling. Finally, see if you can describe what determines the intensity of that emotion.

☐ **Happiness**

☐ **Sadness**

☐ **Fear**

☐ **Disgust**

☐ **Anger**

☐ **Surprise**

What's determining the intensity of these emotions I feel?

My Hero to My Zero

BPD tends to cause you to see others in extremes, all good (hero) or all bad (zero), which can degrade your relationships over time. Describe the person, or people, in your life that you feel are heroes (idealized others) and zeros (devalued others) and write out the characteristics that make them that way (that is, things they say or do).

My Hero	My Zero

Triggers to My Hostility and Aggression

Managing aggressive responses can be one of the hardest things to do when you have BPD. What are some of the behaviors you engage in when you're angry?

Knowing what triggers these responses gives you insight and choice in how to react. Describe those triggers that drive your aggressive behaviors. These can be thoughts, feelings, situations, and so on.

What's My Worth?

BPD causes you to see yourself in an inaccurate and darker light, which diminishes your worth in your perspective. Explore your worth using the prompts below and be aware of the negative perspective that might creep in.

What actions and activities make me feel worthy?

_____

_____

_____

What do I do well?

_____

_____

_____

What behaviors or situations cause me to doubt my capabilities? Is this doubt always justified?

_____

_____

_____

Depth of Aloneness

Aloneness is that feeling of being disconnected from your past, present, and future. BPD enhances these emotions through distortions of how you see yourself, others, and your world. Describe your aloneness as a start, and we'll confront and overcome this in the next two sections.

Who's in Your Heart

Sometimes we forget to stop and remember the most important people in our life who help us move forward. Write the names of those people you hold in your heart below.

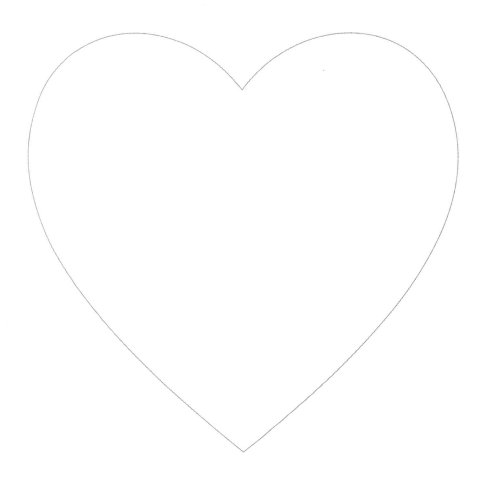

Gathered to Go Forward

As we reach the end of part 1, describe the most salient entries in your journal so far and what you've learned about yourself and your BPD.

Part 2

Surmounting Obstacles to My Growth

Emotions of Growth

What emotions do you feel when you think about growing beyond your BPD and what might be holding you back? Don't edit your thoughts—just let them flow.

Relationship Stifling

What holds you back from having the relationship you want? Is it abandonment or rejection fears, self-doubt, low self-worth, or something else? Fears keep us from growing with our relationships, leading to them outgrowing us. Describe your stifling relationship fears.

Oh, the Things I Do!

Impulsive behaviors are often aimed at breaking down barriers, but maladaptive behaviors tend to raise or solidify them. What are some of your barrier-building behaviors you can bring into awareness, to do differently next time?

Shackles of Thoughts

Beliefs about yourself are powerful influences to control your world or create blocks. What are your three most obstacle-building thoughts? They usually have "can't," "won't," or "will never" in them.

_____

_____

_____

_____

_____

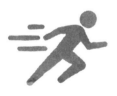

Now imagine yourself free from your thought shackles and replace the "can't," "won't," and "will never" with "I'm able to," "I can do," and "I will do." Then, look inward. How do you feel? Freer and less restricted?

Let's run with this onto the next page!

Keywords of Self-Liberation

Now that you've gotten a taste of your potential, describe it below in as much detail as you can and give yourself three keywords to remind yourself of these feelings.

Keyword #1	Keyword #2	Keyword #3

Hole of Rejection

Rejection can make you feel like you're falling into a bottomless hole and never going to get out. To beat this, you have to confront it. Write the thoughts, feelings, and images connected to your hole of rejection on the lines below. Surmount this by going past it to the next journal entry page.

Steps to Acceptance

Self-acceptance will get you through the hard times and keep you out of the hole of rejection created by your fears. Being kind to yourself is the first step to self-acceptance. And yes, you deserve kindness, especially from yourself. List two things you can do to be kind to yourself. Hint: Use statements of encouragement, such as "Stay strong!" and "Never give up!"

1. _____

_____

2. _____

_____

Your Mind's Eye

Imagine those barriers created by your BPD. These are likely to be your maladaptive beliefs, behaviors, and patterns that disrupt your relationships, job, family, and so on. Perhaps you acted out impulsively or said something you shouldn't have. Put your mind's eye onto paper to increase your awareness by describing each barrier below, as this will help you build insight into it and better control it.

Interrogate Your Abandonment

Abandonment fears can be so intense that you back away or try to avoid them altogether. The problem in doing this is that it makes them stronger. Let's interrogate it, as if it's a thief stealing your freedom, by asking the top five questions below. We're not gonna let this perp get away with it any longer!

1. What created your abandonment? (Think back and don't edit whatever comes up.)

2. When do your abandonment fears present most often?

3. What do you do when your abandonment fears take over?

4. Do others notice when these fears creep up? How are they noticeable? What do you say or do?

5. Whom do you seek support from when these fears take over?

The Manifestation of Your Abandonment

Abandonment fears can set off a pattern that destroys your relationships. Over time, these become second nature, and you don't notice them until the damage has manifested and you feel it's your destiny to always be in relationships that fail. Just as you interrogated it, let's inspect how this shows up. Describe how your abandonment manifests in your relationships.

Abandonment Repair

After a rupture in your relationships that was driven by your abandonment fears, what do you do to repair it and what could you do in the future to avoid the rupture in the first place?

_____

_____

_____

_____

_____

_____

_____

_____

_____

_____

_____

_____

_____

_____

_____

Abandonment Reconciliation

You have to envision it before it can become evident and true. Use the space below to describe what you would be like (thoughts, emotions, and behaviors) once you've reconciled your abandonment fears.

Emotional Autopilot

Emotions build quickly and can shroud your ability to see the world as it is; instead, you see it as your BPD wants you to see it. Describe the who, what, when, and how your emotions push you into autopilot. Doing this will help you catch it when it starts and see it when you're in the throes of autopilot.

Loneliness, Detachment, and Fear

Two things that most harm relationships are loneliness and detachment. Many times you may feel emotions that prompt engagement in behaviors that encourage your loneliness and detachment without your even knowing it. Write out what you can do to resist engaging in detachment behaviors when you feel lonely in your relationship.

Embracing My Truth

Being true to yourself is acting according to your beliefs and doing what you think is right for you. Write out three things you can do to be true to yourself and who you want to be, beyond your BPD.

1. ....
....
....

2. ....
....
....

3. ....
....
....

Surviving Your BPD

What are some lessons you've learned from your BPD on how to survive it and control it? Your first instinct may be to think "nothing," but that's your BPD talking. Use your voice and authentic self to recall the skills and lessons you learned to survive.

From Hate to Love

Make a list on the left of the hateful words that pop into your head that your BPD says to you. On the right, write loving words that help you go forward, embrace your true self, and inspire yourself to live your life differently.

Hateful   **Loving**

Relationship Bonds

Draw the web that's formed by your most important relationships. You'll be at the center, and those most important to you—people, pets, or objects—will surround you. Identify how strong each bond is by changing the way you draw each line. Use a simple line, or string, to represent bonds that are

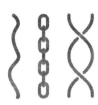

more easily broken. Use a chain to represent bonds that are strong but may degrade, just as chains rust over time. And use a double-helix to represent your strongest and most enduring bonds, just as a chemical is an adhesive that never erodes.

Feels Good

What are three healthy things you can do for yourself to feel good? Examples include making a positive song playlist, preparing a healthy meal or decadent dessert to share, attending a yoga class, and so on.

1.

2.

3.

Things Get Better

You've made it through many hard days and difficult times. Write a letter of encouragement that reminds you things get better, even during tough times. If you have trouble doing this, ask a friend or therapist to help you write it. I've helped you get started.

Dear me, myself, and I:

I've made it through hard days and tough times because...

_____

_____

_____

_____

_____

_____

_____

_____

Favorite Person at a Distance

The favorite person (FP) relationship can evoke a lot of negative feelings. When you feel distant from your FP, you may feel abandoned, unseen, or otherwise unimportant. This is your BPD tricking you into being dependent and helpless, but you're not. Write three things you can do to help yourself feel more confident and independent, whatever your relationship is with your FP at any point in time.

1. _____

_____

2. _____

_____

3. _____

_____

Rise Above the Hurt

There may be times when your partner says or does things that upset you and you feel hurt and confused. This is prime time for your BPD to manipulate you and seemingly shatter your world. In these instances, you have to say and do things for yourself to rise above the hurt.

Write a confidence-building self-statement that shifts your focus to the positive. I've listed some examples for you below.

"Focus on the possibilities instead of the obstacles."

"Embrace the excitement of potential rather than the fear of failure."

"Let optimism be your compass, not anxiety."

My confidence self-statement is:

_____

_____

Find an image or a song, or both, that speak empowerment to you. Make this your cellphone lock screen, or print it out and put it on your bathroom mirror.

Setting My Path

Every goal is accomplished by a first step. Write a goal for tomorrow for yourself and one first step to put you on the path to achieving it. After you do, put that glorious checkmark in the box (that always feels so good).

Goal for tomorrow:

My first steps:

☐ Done!

True Thoughts

Take a deep breath in and think about the negative self-statements you say to yourself. Now, breathe out, and with that, imagine the negative floating out. You're now left with the positives that are often shrouded by the negatives. Write your positive thoughts below and refer to this page often: several times a day is ideal.

Releasing the Pain of Self-Stigma

Self-stigma is made up of the negative attitudes you have about yourself due to having BPD, or other mental health issues. This self-stigma is often paired with painful emotions, but if we lessen one, we lessen the other. Write the positive emotions that help you feel honorable and good about who you are.

A Caring Ear

Think of a positive and healthy person in your life you've been meaning to reach out to. This could be a friend, therapist, or anyone who cares about you and your well-being. Write out below what you want to tell them.

Anti-Fear Movement

Think about those things you wish you would do to help yourself feel better and stronger but are reluctant to get started on out of fear, or talk yourself out of them. This can be working out, talking to an old friend, making and eating healthy recipes, and so on. List five things you're going to include in your anti-fear movement below and do them over the next week.

1. _____

_____

2. _____

_____

3. _____

_____

4. _____

_____

5. _____

_____

Two-Way Empathy

Empathy is a two-way street for sure. The best way to get empathy is to give it. Write the names of three people and how you can show them empathy the next time you're interacting with them. Think about how that person is feeling based on what they're saying and their facial expressions.

Insults

When you feel insulted, you likely go from 0 to 100 in no time. This can blind you to options to de-escalate the conflict and use adaptive strategies to control the situation. Below, write the top three insults that tend to provoke you and what you can do differently to control yourself and the situation.

Calming Conflicted Close Relationships

Many relationship conflicts come out of impulse and fear, followed by regret and even more intense fear. Recognizing and planning your response will help keep you in control and calm the conflict. Think of a recent relationship conflict and write out how you would handle it differently next time.

Risk-Removal Machine

Your BPD often drives you to engage in risky behaviors without a second thought. Replacing risky behaviors like acting out, using substances, and so on with adaptive ones will lessen the hold BPD has over you. Think about the last time you engaged in risky self-destructive behaviors. Describe what you will do differently next time.

Picture of Panic

When your anxiety reaches a tipping point and your brain and body become overwhelmed, you experience panic. This is often accompanied by mental images that throw gas on the fire. Extinguish it by replacing those images with empowering and calming ones. You can describe them or draw them in the space provided.

Peaceful Destinations

If you could go someplace where your BPD couldn't find you, where would you go and what would it be like? What would you be like? What worries, fears, and thoughts would you leave behind?

Distant but Connected

Transitional objects are those things that help you feel connected to something or someone else—a keychain, a stuffed animal, and so on. They can be powerful and comforting tools when your favorite person isn't available or nearby. Describe your object or paste a picture of it here and describe how it makes you feel.

Pushing People Away

Describe what you do to push people away.

_____

_____

_____

_____

_____

What can you do to resist this urge or tendency?

_____

_____

_____

_____

_____

Perfidious Pessimism

Your BPD wants you to fixate on the possible negatives, so that's all you see. Your pessimism is untrustworthy, so let's kick it right out by seeing the positives in a situation you thought was only negative. Describe what you envision.

Emotional Recovery

When you're flooded by negative emotions it's hard to see and feel that you can and will recover. You can speed this up by flooding yourself with positives, like eating something yummy, doing something silly, or watching something funny. Describe what you're going to do next time to emotionally recover quicker.

Fills Me Up

Think of an important relationship in your life. Fill in the cup below to represent how full you feel in this relationship.

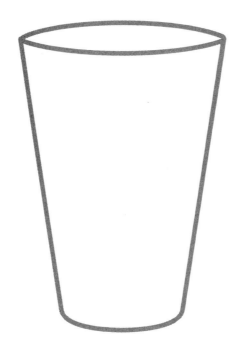

Describe why you filled it as much or as little as you did.

_____

_____

Decisions Against Dependency

Your BPD makes you believe you can't do anything alone, but there are many things you can do without approval from others. List the healthy things you can do for yourself, by yourself, without worrying about approval from others.

Here's What I Think!

It's better out than in, so write what you think about your BPD and the world it's created for you. Getting this out helps you see it and change it. Don't forget to do part 2 on the next page.

Rethinking What I Thunk

Review what you wrote for the previous journal entry. Now describe what you think you and your world would be like without your BPD's contamination.

_____

_____

_____

_____

_____

_____

_____

_____

_____

_____

_____

When I'm a Live Wire

What are the emotions that overwhelm you in an instant? These are the ones that make you feel like a live wire, highly energized and out of control. These are likely tied to your BPD and past experiences. Identify and describe your live wire emotions to raise your awareness and self-control.

Emotion	What It Feels Like

Time-Out Time

When you're triggered, especially in conversations with a partner, it's really hard to recognize the importance of taking a step back and giving yourself and your partner a time-out to process what is going on. Describe the last argument you had with your partner and how a time-out would have helped. You can even share this with your partner, if you'd like.

Non-Self-Inflicting

When you're overwhelmed, you're more likely to go to those old maladaptive self-harm behaviors. This creates a very painful and deleterious habit. You can break that habit by giving yourself behavioral alternatives and finding non-self-inflicting behaviors, such as throwing tennis balls at a wall as hard as you can, doing a plank until you just can't anymore, screaming as loud as you can into a pillow, and so on. List your non-self-inflicting behaviors in the lines provided. And do them until they're a habit.

From Them

Write a letter to yourself that you wish an important person in your life would have written to you. This helps you raise your awareness of the good parts of you, the needs you have, and your wants. Keep it as positive as you can, and even though the other person didn't write it, it's still out there in the world, in your journal—and that's important!

Dear _____,

_____

_____

_____

_____

_____

_____

_____

_____

All-Too-Familiar Pain

It may be loneliness, abandonment, emptiness, or another painful emotion you feel so often that it's become a part of you. Identify what other aspects of your life you want to embrace instead of this pain, or envision how your life might unfold without the presence of this all-too-familiar pain.

Heard but Not Listened To

So many conversations are people hearing you but not listening. Write out those words, phrases, and behaviors that help you feel listened to and understood by those you're in a relationship with; it doesn't have to be a romantic one.

Spit Out the Venom

Over the years, your BPD had filled you with venom. This is from being mistreated, ignored, disrespected, and so on. Holding on to the venom has poisoned you against yourself, making it hard to manage and control your BPD. Describe those venomous instances here. Then, I want you to think of each one and spit them out—literally: outside or into the sink is preferred. It's always better out than in.

Invisible to All Others

A common thought is that you'll be rejected, then invisible, or unknown, to the people in your life if they knew what was going on inside of you. What do you want others to know about your life that helps you feel recognized and present?

_____

_____

_____

_____

_____

_____

_____

_____

_____

_____

_____

Definitely Useful

Your BPD wants you to feel empty and worthless, so it has a place to stay inside you. Use the space to identify those things about you that confirm your worth. These don't have to be things for others to notice; they can just be for you.

Relationship of Want over Need

Dependency is created when we feel we *need* to be with someone else. Relationships blossom when we *want* to be with someone, we have a say in that, and we can appreciate the true desire to be present in it. What are the things in a relationship that make you *want* to be in it, over needing to be in it?

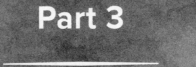

Part 3

Paving My Empowered Future

Emotionally Controlled Future

When you think about your past compared to what you want in your future, which emotions assisted in successful outcomes and which didn't? List them below to help you keep them in awareness as you grow forward.

Successful Emotions   **Destructive Emotions**

Tomorrow's Love

If you could create the perfect relationship, what would it entail? What emotions, behaviors, and strategies to overcome challenges would you and that other person use? Write them out below so you know what to look for and encourage.

Eyeing Your Future

Below is the window for you to your future. As you draw it, focus on the things you want to help you grow beyond your BPD and the things that are indicative of a healthy and happy future.

Thinking About Tomorrow

Describe your future using only positive terms. Examine what your self-statements would be, your job, relationships, and other aspects of your life.

Making Them True

When you read your previous journal entry, how do you feel? Describe those emotions that came up that were the most intense. What can you do to make this future true for you?

Relationship Hope

Think about the relationships that mean the most to you in your life. Do they feel hopeful or hopeless? Describe what makes them seem this way. Are they things about you, another person, or both?

Hopeless	Hopeful

Building on Hope

Looking back at your previous journal entry, what can you do to increase your hopefulness and decrease your hopelessness?

Decrease Hopelessness Behaviors	Increase Hopefulness Behaviors

Wiener-to-Winner Thinking

The most successful people in history all had one thing in common: they had winning thinking. They believed they could do and achieve the things they wanted and needed in their life. Use the space below to turn your wiener (negative) thinking into winning thinking.

Wiener Thinking		Winner Thinking
	→	
	→	
	→	
	→	

Emotional Inventory

Every system needs an inventory check, and your mental health is no different. Following are some common intense emotions people with BPD tend to experience—but one size doesn't fit all. I have left some blank for you to write in your own. Next to each emotion, rate it from 0 (I haven't felt it the last two weeks) to 10 (I can't stop feeling it and it's hard to control).

Rating	Emotion	Rating	Emotion
	Abandonment		Anger/rage
	Emptiness		Despair
	Self-contempt		Fear

"Over" Is Not Forever

When relationships end, it can feel like you'll be alone forever and that you're so broken you broke your relationship. Write a note reminding yourself that when a relationship is over, it doesn't mean all relationships are forever over for you. Let your optimism come through, not your BPD.

Your Future Brain/Body

What you do today impacts your tomorrow in a positive or negative way. List those things you're going to do today to enhance your brain and body wellness.

Abandon Abandonment Fears

Your thoughts help dictate and control your fears of abandonment. What are the thoughts that help you feel connected to your world and the people in it? These may be encouraging thoughts about your worth, appearance, intelligence, and so on.

_____

_____

_____

_____

_____

_____

_____

_____

_____

_____

_____

_____

Intoxicating Shame

Shame is often an emotional precursor to alcohol and drug use, and it can become a familiar, painful partner. Describe your future without the pain of shame. What does this freedom—from painful emotions and shame-fueled substance use—look like and feel like? How does it help you grow in your future?

Relationship of Substances

Drug and alcohol dependence builds slowly, and as it does you develop a maladaptive relationship with it. Like all unhealthy relationships, you must purge them from your future. To do this you need to map out steps forward. I've started those steps for you below. Every success starts with a first step.

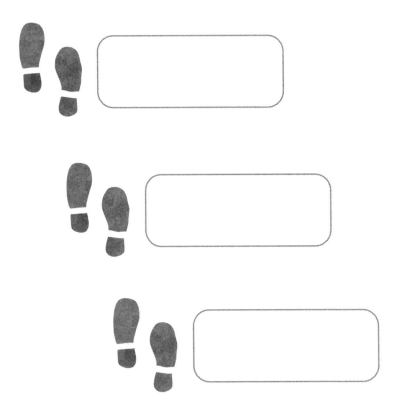

Adaptive Avoidance

Access is the #1 issue you have to maintain control of when you start on the road to a future of sobriety. Taking an inventory of where you consume substances most often and how to avoid consumption is an invaluable first step.

Where I Consume Most	How I Can Avoid Consumption

The Intoxicated or Sober Me

Describe how you see yourself when you're under the influence, and then describe when you're not. Circle which one you want to take with you in the future.

Intoxicated Me

_____

_____

_____

_____

Sober Me

_____

_____

_____

_____

Boredom Battle

When you're bored, your mind likely wanders to dark places. Battling this means preparing to push back on your boredom. This can be spending time with friends, watching something funny, going to a new place, and so on. Write your targets for the coming day or week—the events or situations that you know will cause boredom—and your battle plan for how you'll handle them.

Missing Pieces

Think about your past relationships—what was missing in them? Was it honesty, openness, affection, and so on? Describe here what your relationships would look like with these pieces filled in.

_____

_____

_____

_____

_____

_____

_____

_____

_____

_____

_____

_____

How I Show Love

List five ways you will openly show people in your life that you love them with no strings attached. Remember, showing love is giving to give, not giving to get.

1.

2.

3.

4.

5.

Repaired

If you were a robot and went in for repairs, what would need to be fixed and how would it change your life going forward?

_____

_____

_____

_____

What steps do you need to take to make these repairs?

_____

_____

_____

_____

Caged Worries

Caging your worries means that you've learned containment strategies, and they're not running your life anymore. How have you caged your worries since you started this journal?

_____

_____

_____

_____

_____

_____

_____

_____

_____

_____

_____

_____

_____

Showing Your Love

Visualization leads to realization! Imagine yourself one year from now and how you'll be expressing your love and caring for those most important in your life. Describe what's in your mind's eye.

Daily Determination

Change is never easy because it takes focus and practice. What adaptive behaviors are you going to do starting today to help you push back on your BPD and grow in a positive way?

Thoughts Aren't Everything

What we think is important, but it's not the only way we can change; our emotions and behaviors count, too. What behaviors and emotions can you employ to change or lessen the impact of your BPD in your life today?

Emotional Refuel

Controlling your BPD and its influence on you takes energy, and a lot of it. Keeping your fuel tank full—replenishing yourself with rest and self-care— is a critical step. What emotions can you harness to help you keep your tank full?

Communication Clarity

Below are steps to help you communicate in a more effective way. Review the steps below and write how you will implement each step in your relationship to keep it calm and cool.

Viewpoint: See the issue from the other person's perspective.

_____

_____

_____

Feelings: What feelings are making it hard for you to see their viewpoint?

_____

_____

_____

Convey compassion: How can you communicate kindness while getting your message across?

_____

_____

_____

Explosion Prevention

Write out what you think and feel just prior to acting out impulsively and what you can do differently. Remember many of the strategies you've learned from this journal.

My Thoughtful Inventory

Take an inventory of your negative and positive self-statements. Positive statements encourage growth, so it's important to have more optimistic and encouraging ones compared to harmful ones.

Negative Self-Statements	Positive Self-Statements

BPD Creep

"BPD creep" is when your old emotions reemerge for no *obvious* reasons. It's the word "obvious" that makes it so you have to explore this experience and find the triggers that prompt your BPD to creep back into your life. Write out the clues that can help you pinpoint the creep.

What's your stress level today?

What are your fears and what's causing them to intensify?

What's making you feel unbalanced?

Relationship Risk

Impulsive urges and responsive behavior can put your important relationships at risk. Describe your impulsive urges or the risky behaviors you're contemplating, then ask yourself, "Is it worth it?"

Is it worth it? ☐ YES ☐ NO

Countdown to Self-Destruction

You've learned so much to manage and control your BPD, but this does not mean those old maladaptive beliefs, behaviors, and patterns won't tempt you from time to time. Writing them out will stop your countdown clock and put you back in control.

Painful Memories

Managing BPD is difficult and it's an ongoing process, and there will be times when old memories may come back. Keeping them inside only gives them more power. Weaken them by writing them out and the emotions and behaviors associated with them. Release them and free yourself.

It's Okay to Be Upset

Your BPD tells you you're wrong to feel upset or angry. These emotions are normal and not wrong. It's what we do with them that creates problems. Write out what you will do in the future that is not destructive when you feel upset and angry.

Mastering My Relationship

What makes you feel present and at peace in your relationship? If you're not in one right now, imagine the things that would, as these help you identify the things you want out of your relationships.

My Good Deeds

You've likely forgotten all the good things you've done in your past that have helped others and yourself to grow and do well. No one does only bad things. Write out your good deeds as a thoughtful reminder to yourself.

You Can Get Some Satisfaction

Write out three things you're going to do tomorrow to help yourself feel satisfied and grateful.

My Emotional Needs

Write out what you can do to nurture your positive emotional needs. This can be a mindfulness activity, engaging in exercise, or writing more in your journal.

_____

_____

_____

_____

_____

_____

_____

_____

_____

_____

_____

_____

_____

_____

_____

Who's Got My Back?

Write down up to three people in your life who have your back. These are people you feel you can count on when you need help.

1. _____

   _____

2. _____

   _____

3. _____

   _____

Picture Your Way to Peace

All our behavior is subsequent to some thought or image in our mind. You can manage your tendency to act out toward yourself or others by changing this mental picture from one of violence to one of calm. Describe or draw your peaceful picture in the space provided. Work to cement this image in your brain to promote a calmer future.

No More Self-Rejection

Self-acceptance starts with tolerant thoughts about yourself and your behavior. Your BPD has likely encouraged you to be intolerant, but it's time to add balance to your thoughts and be less self-rejecting. Write thoughts that are more self-accepting and tolerant of who you are and the things you do.

Self-Comforting

Your BPD told you that only negative emotions mattered, which kept you in a state of vigilance and fear. Write out those emotions that help you feel comforted and what you can do to encourage those emotions.

Lasting Love

Creating lasting love entails friendship, patience, communication, managing conflicts, and relationship encouragement. Describe how these things are or are not present in your current relationship. (Be sure to check out the second part of this entry on the next page.)

Creating Lasting Love

Review your journal entry from the previous page and write out what you can do going forward to foster friendship, patience, communication, conflict management, and relationship encouragement.

So You Think ...

You should be proud of yourself for getting this far in your journal. Write how this journal has helped you manage and control your maladaptive BPD thoughts.

Living Through Truth

When we live in a genuine way, we recognize ourselves, take responsibility for what we do, and contain fear that would drive us backward. Describe how you're going to live your truth.

Give to Give

Relationships where both partners give to give are ones that are strong and tend to endure. The ones in which partners give to make sure they get something equal or of better value in return are often doomed and toxic to one's growth. Write ways you can give to give in your relationship to nurture it.

Stop Falsely Fighting Yourself

Your BPD tricked you for so long into believing that every thought, feeling, and behavior you had was wrong and demanded that you fight it. Describe what you can do to be gentle, patient, and caring with yourself going forward. Tip: Embrace what you deserve—don't fight it.

Foundation of Emotional Confidence

Being emotionally confident is based upon recognizing that even though you can't control the thoughts that pop into your mind, you have control over how long you focus on them. Below, describe the more helpful thoughts that you can replace popped-in thoughts with and the things you can do to give yourself a sense of emotional control and confidence.

References

Gunderson, John G., Robert L. Stout, Thomas H. McGlashan, M. Tracie Shea, Leslie C. Morey, Carlos M. Grilo, Mary C. Zanarini, et al. 2011. "Ten-Year Course of Borderline Personality Disorder: Psychopathology and Function from the Collaborative Longitudinal Personality Disorders Study." *Archives of General Psychiatry* 68, no. 8: 827–837.

Zanarini, Mary C., Frances R. Frankenburg, John Hennen, D. Bradford Reich, and Kenneth R. Silk. 2005. "Psychosocial Functioning of Borderline Patients and Axis II Comparison Subjects Followed Prospectively for Six Years." *Journal of Personality Disorders* 19, no. 1: 19–29.

Daniel J. Fox, PhD, is a personality disorder expert, and award-winning author of several books, including *The Borderline Personality Disorder Workbook* and *Complex Borderline Personality Disorder*. For more than twenty years, he has been diagnosing and successfully treating clients in his private practice, as well as at universities and in state and federal prison systems.

Also by Daniel J. Fox

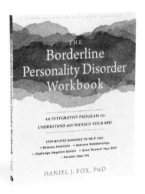

ISBN 978-1684032730 / US $24.95

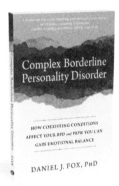

ISBN 978-1684038558 / US $18.95

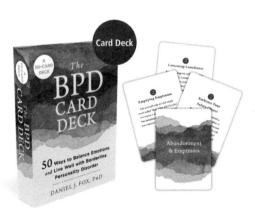

ISBN 978-1648480843 / US $18.95

🌱 new**harbinger**publications

1-800-748-6273 / newharbinger.com